START HEALTH CONSCIOUS LIVING TODAY

With thought provoking QUOTES that will move you to take action towards better health

Health Conscious Living Journal

By Martha Walters

This journal is intended to encourage the reader to choose better health and for no other purpose.

All quotes are the express opinion of the author, unless otherwise indicated, and should be taken as such.

ISBN-13: 978-1540878557

ISBN-10: 1540878554

www.todayichooselife.com

This Journal is a gift to:

_____

Message:

_____
_____
_____
_____
_____

From:

_____

A change in you = A change in the next generation

Introduction

Good health is one of the most valuable things that a human possesses, and without it, you have nothing.

How many dreams have been shattered, changed, put on hold, lost, or even worse, how many lives gone prematurely because of unexpected illness that led to death? The question is, could it all have been prevented? We do not always know the answers to these questions; however, we do know our bodies need optimal conditions to thrive. This includes good nutrition, movement, quality rest, and stress management to name a few. Live foods, foods that are in their natural state, and have not been altered, for example, are required in order to promote life. The opposite is true. If we eat too much dead foods or foods depleted of nutrients, it will produce sickness and possibly leading to premature death.

Don't sabotage your future and your dreams. Live according to your future plans. Without good health, you may not have the opportunity to fulfill your dreams.

How To Use This Journal

Use this journal to record your plan of action for better health or to record your progress if you are dealing with a health crisis. The quote on each page will motivate you and awaken your consciousness to care for your body so you can follow your dreams and enjoy those you love.

This journal was written with the idea that everyone should pay attention to their health and not wait until sickness strikes. After reading the quotes in this journal, you will think differently about your health, and how sickness could impact your life.

There are things we do not have control over, how we care for our body is not one of them.

Start your health journey today and be in health as your soul prospers! [III John 1:2]

-Your partner in Health, Martha Walters

My health journey   Date_____

_____

_____

_____

_____

_____

_____

_____

_____

_____

_____

_____

_____

_____

_____

_____

_____

_____

_____

Beloved, I wish above all things that thou mayest prosper and be in *HEALTH*, even as thy *SOUL* prospereth. **III John 1:2**

My health journey

_____

_____

_____

_____

_____

_____

_____

_____

_____

_____

_____

_____

_____

_____

_____

_____

_____

_____

LIFE and *DEATH* have been set before you, blessing and cursing: therefore *CHOOSE LIFE*, that both you and your seed may live. **Deuteronomy 30:19**

My health journey

_____

_____

_____

_____

_____

_____

_____

_____

_____

_____

_____

_____

_____

_____

_____

_____

_____

_____

Every day that you live, is a chance that you have been given to choose life.

My health journey   Date_____

_____

_____

_____

_____

_____

_____

_____

_____

_____

_____

_____

_____

_____

_____

_____

_____

_____

_____

How you take care of your body, is preparing you for tomorrow.
The question is, "Are you preparing for *SICKNESS OR HEALTH*?

My health journey

Date_____

_____

_____

_____

_____

_____

_____

_____

_____

_____

_____

_____

_____

_____

_____

_____

_____

_____

_____

I will treat my body right because I *LOVE LIFE*.

My health journey Date_____

_____

_____

_____

_____

_____

_____

_____

_____

_____

_____

_____

_____

_____

_____

_____

_____

_____

_____

_____

QUALITY OF LIFE is a choice that starts early in life and will produce dividends.

My health journey Date_____

_____

_____

_____

_____

_____

_____

_____

_____

_____

_____

_____

_____

_____

_____

_____

_____

_____

_____

On a scale of 1-10, how important is *BEING HEALTHY* to you?
Only you can answer this question.

My health journey   Date_____

_____

_____

_____

_____

_____

_____

_____

_____

_____

_____

_____

_____

_____

_____

_____

_____

_____

_____

How much is your health worth to you? Without good health, you have nothing.

My health journey

Date_____

_____

_____

_____

_____

_____

_____

_____

_____

_____

_____

_____

_____

_____

_____

_____

_____

_____

_____

What you're feeding your mind, body, and spirit, may cut your life short, preventing you from reaching your *FULL POTENTIAL.*

My health journey

_____

_____

_____

_____

_____

_____

_____

_____

_____

_____

_____

_____

_____

_____

_____

_____

Don't *SABOTAGE* your future by choosing to live an un-healthy lifestyle.

My health journey

_____

_____

_____

_____

_____

_____

_____

_____

_____

_____

_____

_____

_____

_____

_____

_____

_____

_____

_____

Make being healthy a priority in your life. Nothing else will matter without it.

My health journey

_____

_____

_____

_____

_____

_____

_____

_____

_____

_____

_____

_____

_____

_____

_____

_____

_____

GOOD HEALTH happens not by chance, but by choice.

My health journey

_____

_____

_____

_____

_____

_____

_____

_____

_____

_____

_____

_____

_____

_____

_____

_____

_____

_____

_____

Someone out there **NEEDS YOU**. Be healthy.

My health journey

Date_____

_____

_____

_____

_____

_____

_____

_____

_____

_____

_____

_____

_____

_____

_____

_____

_____

_____

Where health consciousness *BEGINS,* illness will *END.*

My health journey

Date_____

_____

_____

_____

_____

_____

_____

_____

_____

_____

_____

_____

_____

_____

_____

_____

_____

_____

_____

_____

_____

_____

We owe it to our loved ones to be healthy.

My health journey   Date_____

_____

_____

_____

_____

_____

_____

_____

_____

_____

_____

_____

_____

_____

_____

_____

_____

_____

Being healthy should be all about changing your family tree.
Choose health!

My health journey

Only 20% of your illness is *DNA*; 80% is choice.

My health journey

_____

_____

_____

_____

_____

_____

_____

_____

_____

_____

_____

_____

_____

_____

_____

_____

_____

Today, a 1/4 of what you eat feeds your body; the other 3/4 of what you eat feeds the doctor's pocket.

My health journey

_____

_____

_____

_____

_____

_____

_____

_____

_____

_____

_____

_____

_____

_____

_____

_____

_____

_____

_____

Change *YOUR DNA* by changing your eating habits.

My health journey   Date_____

_____

_____

_____

_____

_____

_____

_____

_____

_____

_____

_____

_____

_____

_____

_____

_____

_____

_____

"Health is not valued till sickness comes"- Dr. Thomas Fuller.

My health journey

_____

_____

_____

_____

_____

_____

_____

_____

_____

_____

_____

_____

_____

_____

_____

_____

_____

_____

_____

_____

Your eating habits should be *ALIGNED* with your future plans.

My health journey

_____

_____

_____

_____

_____

_____

_____

_____

_____

_____

_____

_____

_____

_____

_____

_____

_____

_____

Choose to be healthy today. Your future self, will thank you.

My health journey   Date_____

_____

_____

_____

_____

_____

_____

_____

_____

_____

_____

_____

_____

_____

_____

_____

_____

_____

_____

The best way to *PREDICT* your health, is to *CREATE IT.*

My health journey   Date_____

_____

_____

_____

_____

_____

_____

_____

_____

_____

_____

_____

_____

_____

_____

_____

_____

_____

When you could, you didn't. Now you want to, and you can't.

My health journey

_____

_____

_____

_____

_____

_____

_____

_____

_____

_____

_____

_____

_____

_____

_____

_____

_____

_____

Worrying won't change anything. Things will eventually work themselves out. Just **BE HAPPY**! It will do your body good.

My health journey

_____

_____

_____

_____

_____

_____

_____

_____

_____

_____

_____

_____

_____

_____

_____

_____

_____

Life is *GOOD*; take the time to *ENJOY* it.

My health journey   Date_____

_____

_____

_____

_____

_____

_____

_____

_____

_____

_____

_____

_____

_____

_____

_____

_____

_____

_____

Don't just wish to be healthy. You have to work at it with intention.

My health journey

You have **ONE BODY** to navigate this earth; **TAKE CARE OF IT**, and it will take care of you.

My health journey   Date_____

_____

_____

_____

_____

_____

_____

_____

_____

_____

_____

_____

_____

_____

_____

_____

_____

_____

_____

Your current health reflects the *CHOICES* you have made.
Different results, require different choices.

My health journey   Date_____

_____

_____

_____

_____

_____

_____

_____

_____

_____

_____

_____

_____

_____

_____

_____

_____

_____

_____

Being healthy is not easy, but it is worth it. Think about all the
REASONS WHY.

My health journey   Date_____

_____

_____

_____

_____

_____

_____

_____

_____

_____

_____

_____

_____

_____

_____

_____

_____

_____

_____

Think about who may suffer if you leave this earth
PREMATURELY.

My health journey

_____

_____

_____

_____

_____

_____

_____

_____

_____

_____

_____

_____

_____

_____

_____

_____

_____

_____

Choose to live a *HEALTHY* lifestyle today. Your *FAMILY* will *BENEFIT* from it.

My health journey Date_____

_____

_____

_____

_____

_____

_____

_____

_____

_____

_____

_____

_____

_____

_____

_____

_____

_____

_____

Someone is *DEPENDING ON YOU* to be healthy. Choose to be healthy today.

My health journey

_____

_____

_____

_____

_____

_____

_____

_____

_____

_____

_____

_____

_____

_____

_____

_____

_____

_____

_____

If you *LOVE* your *CHILDREN*, be healthy for them.

My health journey   Date_____

_____

_____

_____

_____

_____

_____

_____

_____

_____

_____

_____

_____

_____

_____

_____

_____

_____

_____

_____

_____

Children are your most *PRECIOUS POSSESSION*. A health change in you = a change in the next generation.

My health journey   Date_____

_____

_____

_____

_____

_____

_____

_____

_____

_____

_____

_____

_____

_____

_____

_____

_____

_____

Children mimic what they see. Eat healthy, and they will follow.

My health journey

Children benefit from the love of their *GRANDPARENTS*. Choose to be around for them.

My health journey　　　　　　　　　　Date＿＿＿＿＿＿＿＿

_____

_____

_____

_____

_____

_____

_____

_____

_____

_____

_____

_____

_____

_____

_____

Your children are planning on you being there for their wedding.
Choose health!

My health journey

_____

_____

_____

_____

_____

_____

_____

_____

_____

_____

_____

_____

_____

_____

_____

_____

_____

_____

It took more than a day to put it on. It will take more than a day to take it off. Go easy on yourself.

My health journey　　　　　　　　　　Date_____

_____

_____

_____

_____

_____

_____

_____

_____

_____

_____

_____

_____

_____

_____

_____

_____

_____

Iron rusts from disuse; *STAGNANT WATER* loses its purity and
in cold weather become frozen; even so inaction sap the vigor of
the mind.- Leonardo da Vinci

My health journey

_____

_____

_____

_____

_____

_____

_____

_____

_____

_____

_____

_____

_____

_____

_____

_____

_____

MOVE, MOVE, MOVE. You can feel sore today, or you can feel sorry tomorrow. You Choose!

My health journey

_____

_____

_____

_____

_____

_____

_____

_____

_____

_____

_____

_____

_____

_____

_____

_____

_____

_____

Don't let your body tell you how you feel; rather, you tell it how to feel, and *IT WILL LISTEN.*

My health journey

_____

_____

_____

_____

_____

_____

_____

_____

_____

_____

_____

_____

_____

_____

_____

_____

_____

_____

_____

_____

Where your mind goes, your body will follow. *THINK RIGHT.*

My health journey   Date_____

_____

_____

_____

_____

_____

_____

_____

_____

_____

_____

_____

_____

_____

_____

_____

_____

_____

I feed my mind happy thoughts because they promote good health.

My health journey

_____

_____

_____

_____

_____

_____

_____

_____

_____

_____

_____

_____

_____

_____

_____

_____

_____

_____

Some things you do not have control over, however, what you
CHOOSE TO EAT is not one of them.

My health journey

_____

_____

_____

_____

_____

_____

_____

_____

_____

_____

_____

_____

_____

_____

_____

_____

_____

_____

BALANCE and *SELF-CONTROL* are two important companions to your health journey.

My health journey

_____

_____

_____

_____

_____

_____

_____

_____

_____

_____

_____

_____

_____

_____

_____

_____

As I gain knowledge of how to care for my body, I choose to
APPLY IT.

My health journey

_____

_____

_____

_____

_____

_____

_____

_____

_____

_____

_____

_____

_____

_____

_____

You are not able to change your *HEIGHT*, but you can change your *WAIST LINE*.

My health journey

Date_____

_____

_____

_____

_____

_____

_____

_____

_____

_____

_____

_____

_____

_____

_____

_____

_____

_____

_____

I will do my part towards living a healthy lifestyle.

My health journey   Date_____

_____

_____

_____

_____

_____

_____

_____

_____

_____

_____

_____

_____

_____

_____

_____

_____

Is your *UNHEALTHY* behavior worth the suffering you may endure later?

My health journey   Date_____

_____

_____

_____

_____

_____

_____

_____

_____

_____

_____

_____

_____

_____

_____

_____

_____

_____

I realize that what I sow I will grow, so I choose to sow towards
my good health.

My health journey

_____

_____

_____

_____

_____

_____

_____

_____

_____

_____

_____

_____

_____

_____

_____

_____

_____

_____

If you could **_TURN BACK TIME_**, what unhealthy behaviors would you change? Change them now!

My health journey

_____

_____

_____

_____

_____

_____

_____

_____

_____

_____

_____

_____

_____

_____

_____

_____

_____

I choose to live a healthy lifestyle today, so I will not have to live
with regrets tomorrow.

My health journey   Date_____

_____

_____

_____

_____

_____

_____

_____

_____

_____

_____

_____

_____

_____

_____

_____

_____

_____

RADIANT HEALTH is the result of a happy and *CONTENT MIND.*

My health journey　　　　　　　　Date_____

_____

_____

_____

_____

_____

_____

_____

_____

_____

_____

_____

_____

_____

_____

_____

_____

_____

_____

HAPPY people are healthy people, and *HEALTHY* people are happy people.

My health journey   Date_____

_____

_____

_____

_____

_____

_____

_____

_____

_____

_____

_____

_____

_____

_____

_____

_____

_____

Do not spend your *LIFE WORKING* to acquire material goods at the expense of your health. You may end up spending the rest of your days trying to regain *YOUR HEALTH.*

My health journey

_____

_____

_____

_____

_____

_____

_____

_____

_____

_____

_____

_____

_____

_____

_____

_____

_____

He who **NEGLECTS** his health trying to gain material wealth, **IS NOT WISE.** He might not be around to enjoy it.

My health journey

_____

_____

_____

_____

_____

_____

_____

_____

_____

_____

_____

_____

_____

_____

_____

_____

_____

_____

_____

HEALTH and *WEALTH* should not have to *COMPETE.*
Choose health.

My health journey

_____

_____

_____

_____

_____

_____

_____

_____

_____

_____

_____

_____

_____

_____

_____

_____

_____

_____

_____

My *HEALTH* is more important than *WEALTH*. I will not sacrifice my health for it.

My health journey

_____

_____

_____

_____

_____

_____

_____

_____

_____

_____

_____

_____

_____

_____

_____

What does it *PROFIT* a man if he has *WEALTH* without *HEALTH?*

My health journey

_____

_____

_____

_____

_____

_____

_____

_____

_____

_____

_____

_____

_____

_____

_____

_____

_____

_____

Without my *HEALTH*, I will not be able to enjoy my *WEALTH*.

My health journey   Date_____

_____

_____

_____

_____

_____

_____

_____

_____

_____

_____

_____

_____

_____

_____

_____

_____

_____

I will not allow *MY HEALTH* to compete with my wealth. I put my health *FIRST*.

My health journey   Date_____

_____

_____

_____

_____

_____

_____

_____

_____

_____

_____

_____

_____

_____

_____

_____

_____

_____

_____

_____

Don't be like the individual who said; "I wish I could **TURN BACK TIME"**. Make a change today.

My health journey

Date_____

_____

_____

_____

_____

_____

_____

_____

_____

_____

_____

_____

_____

_____

_____

_____

If you don't take the *TIME* to take care for your body now, you may be forced to do it later.

My health journey   Date_____

_____

_____

_____

_____

_____

_____

_____

_____

_____

_____

_____

_____

_____

_____

_____

_____

_____

TIME and *HEALTH* are two precious assets that you don't recognize and appreciate until they have been depleted - Denis Waitley

My health journey   Date_____

_____

_____

_____

_____

_____

_____

_____

_____

_____

_____

_____

_____

_____

_____

_____

_____

I know I cannot go back in *TIME*, so I choose to be healthy today.

My health journey

_____

_____

_____

_____

_____

_____

_____

_____

_____

_____

_____

_____

_____

_____

_____

_____

_____

_____

_____

Everyone has the same amount of *TIME* in a day. Allocate time to take care of *YOU*. Your body will say, "Thank you"

My health journey   Date_____

_____

_____

_____

_____

_____

_____

_____

_____

_____

_____

_____

_____

_____

_____

_____

_____

You cannot go back in *TIME*. Make your days count for *HEALTH*.

My health journey

_____

_____

_____

_____

_____

_____

_____

_____

_____

_____

_____

_____

_____

_____

_____

_____

_____

_____

Be conscious of *YOUR THOUGHTS,* as they can either make you well, or they can make you sick.

My health journey

_____

_____

_____

_____

_____

_____

_____

_____

_____

_____

_____

_____

_____

_____

_____

The words you speak, frame the world you live in.

My health journey

_____

_____

_____

_____

_____

_____

_____

_____

_____

_____

_____

_____

_____

_____

_____

_____

_____

_____

Your life is a reflection of the sum of your thoughts and your words.

My health journey   Date_____

_____

_____

_____

_____

_____

_____

_____

_____

_____

_____

_____

_____

_____

_____

_____

YOUR WORDS create your world. Death and life are
in the power of *YOUR TONGUE.* Proverbs 18:21

My health journey

_____

_____

_____

_____

_____

_____

_____

_____

_____

_____

_____

_____

_____

_____

_____

_____

_____

I will speak life over my body, because proverbs 18:21 says that
LIFE IS IN MY TONGUE.

My health journey

_____

_____

_____

_____

_____

_____

_____

_____

_____

_____

_____

_____

_____

_____

_____

_____

Your health is a reflection of what you have been saying.
SPEAK HEALTH.

My health journey   Date_____

_____

_____

_____

_____

_____

_____

_____

_____

_____

_____

_____

_____

_____

_____

_____

_____

_____

_____

_____

He who **LOVES LIFE**, let him **RESTRAIN HIS TONGUE** from speaking evil. Psalms 34:13

My health journey   Date_____

_____

_____

_____

_____

_____

_____

_____

_____

_____

_____

_____

_____

_____

_____

_____

_____

What I say is what I *GET*!

My health journey

Date_____

_____

_____

_____

_____

_____

_____

_____

_____

_____

_____

_____

_____

_____

_____

_____

_____

_____

_____

_____

Choose life by *THINKING* the *RIGHT THOUGHTS*, for as a man thinketh in his heart, so is he. Proverbs 23:7

My health journey

Date_____

_____

_____

_____

_____

_____

_____

_____

_____

_____

_____

_____

_____

_____

_____

_____

_____

_____

_____

I will think right thoughts, based on Proverbs 23:7

My health journey

_____

_____

_____

_____

_____

_____

_____

_____

_____

_____

_____

_____

_____

_____

_____

_____

_____

_____

_____

I will watch what I say because I love life.

My health journey   Date_____

_____

_____

_____

_____

_____

_____

_____

_____

_____

_____

_____

_____

_____

_____

_____

_____

Don't wait for a **WAKE-UP-CALL** to begin your health journey.
Start your journey today!

My health journey

Date_____

_____

_____

_____

_____

_____

_____

_____

_____

_____

_____

_____

_____

_____

_____

_____

_____

_____

_____

I begin my health journey *TODAY*.

My health journey

Your body is like a vehicle. A ***WELL MAINTAINED*** vehicle, will take you far.

My health journey

_____

_____

_____

_____

_____

_____

_____

_____

_____

_____

_____

_____

_____

_____

_____

_____

_____

I treat my body like a *LUXURY CAR*. I put the right fuel in it for optimal health.

My health journey

_____

_____

_____

_____

_____

_____

_____

_____

_____

_____

_____

_____

_____

_____

_____

If you think choosing a healthy lifestyle is expensive,
TRY ILLNESS.

My health journey

_____

_____

_____

_____

_____

_____

_____

_____

_____

_____

_____

_____

_____

_____

_____

_____

_____

_____

_____

_____

PREVENTION is less costly in the long run.

My health journey

_____

_____

_____

_____

_____

_____

_____

_____

_____

_____

_____

_____

_____

_____

_____

_____

_____

Pain is your body telling you that it's *TIME TO MAKE A CHANGE*. Don't ignore the signal.

My health journey

_____

_____

_____

_____

_____

_____

_____

_____

_____

_____

_____

_____

_____

_____

_____

_____

_____

_____

_____

HEALTH is not my doctor's *RESPONSIBILITY*, it's my own.

My health journey   Date_____

_____

_____

_____

_____

_____

_____

_____

_____

_____

_____

_____

_____

_____

_____

_____

_____

Your doctor is only practicing medicine. He/she does not have the last word.

My health journey   Date_____

_____

_____

_____

_____

_____

_____

_____

_____

_____

_____

_____

_____

_____

_____

_____

_____

_____

I will take responsibility for my own health by taking care of my body.

My health journey   Date_____

_____

_____

_____

_____

_____

_____

_____

_____

_____

_____

_____

_____

_____

_____

_____

_____

_____

Don't wait for your **DOCTOR** to give you a **BAD REPORT** before you change. Change today!

My health journey

_____

_____

_____

_____

_____

_____

_____

_____

_____

_____

_____

_____

_____

_____

_____

_____

_____

_____

LAUGHTER is as good as *MEDICINE.* Laugh much!
Proverbs 17:22

My health journey   Date_____

_____

_____

_____

_____

_____

_____

_____

_____

_____

_____

_____

_____

_____

_____

_____

_____

I take my *MEDICINE* every day. I laugh much.

My health journey   Date_____

_____

_____

_____

_____

_____

_____

_____

_____

_____

_____

_____

_____

_____

_____

_____

_____

_____

_____

MEDICINE is like a Band-Aid, a temporary solution that only covers up the wound. Deal with the *ROOT* of your issues, in order to heal.

My health journey

_____

_____

_____

_____

_____

_____

_____

_____

_____

_____

_____

_____

_____

_____

_____

_____

_____

_____

_____

Your **BODY** was designed to be in a state of **PEACEFULNESS**.

My health journey   Date_____

_____

_____

_____

_____

_____

_____

_____

_____

_____

_____

_____

_____

_____

_____

_____

_____

_____

_____

Avoid prolonged *STRESS* in your life, It contributes to illness, and it *KILLS.*

My health journey Date_____

_____

_____

_____

_____

_____

_____

_____

_____

_____

_____

_____

_____

_____

_____

_____

_____

Because *STRESS* is the cause of so many *DISEASES*, I choose a stress-free life.

My health journey   Date_____

_____

_____

_____

_____

_____

_____

_____

_____

_____

_____

_____

_____

_____

_____

_____

_____

_____

_____

_____

Do not take *OWNERSHIP* of *SICKNESS*; your condition is subject to *CHANGE*.

My health journey   Date_____

_____

_____

_____

_____

_____

_____

_____

_____

_____

_____

_____

_____

_____

_____

_____

_____

_____

_____

The *OUTCOME* of your *DIAGNOSIS* will depend on how you *RESPOND* to it.

My health journey   Date_____

_____

_____

_____

_____

_____

_____

_____

_____

_____

_____

_____

_____

_____

_____

_____

_____

_____

_____

My condition is subject to *CHANGE* based on my outlook.

My health journey   Date_____

_____

_____

_____

_____

_____

_____

_____

_____

_____

_____

_____

_____

_____

_____

_____

There is *POWER IN NOW*. Waiting for tomorrow maybe too late. Choose to be healthy today!

My health journey

Date_____

_____

_____

_____

_____

_____

_____

_____

_____

_____

_____

_____

_____

_____

_____

_____

_____

_____

_____

Sowing and reaping is a law that's always at work. Allow this law to work for the good of your health. Choose health!

My health journey   Date_____

_____

_____

_____

_____

_____

_____

_____

_____

_____

_____

_____

_____

_____

_____

_____

_____

Choose to live a healthy lifestyle today and *YOU WILL NOT REGRET IT*.

My health journey

Date_____

_____

_____

_____

_____

_____

_____

_____

_____

_____

_____

_____

_____

_____

_____

_____

_____

_____

_____

_____

No more *PROCRASTINATION*. Stop saying that you need to change, and just do it!

My health journey

_____

_____

_____

_____

_____

_____

_____

_____

_____

_____

_____

_____

_____

_____

_____

_____

_____

_____

Take the time to pursue good health. Don't be forced into doing it.

My health journey   Date_____

_____

_____

_____

_____

_____

_____

_____

_____

_____

_____

_____

_____

_____

_____

_____

_____

_____

_____

_____

_____

SAY YES TO LIFE by choosing to eat more foods in their natural state.

My health journey

_____

_____

_____

_____

_____

_____

_____

_____

_____

_____

_____

_____

_____

_____

_____

_____

_____

Crowd out unhealthy foods by replacing them with healthy ones.

My health journey   Date_____

_____

_____

_____

_____

_____

_____

_____

_____

_____

_____

_____

_____

_____

_____

_____

_____

_____

_____

Living in *DIVINE HEALTH*, is better than seeking divine healing.

My health journey

_____

_____

_____

_____

_____

_____

_____

_____

_____

_____

_____

_____

_____

_____

_____

Maintaining your health is easier to do than trying to regain it.

My health journey

_____

_____

_____

_____

_____

_____

_____

_____

_____

_____

_____

_____

_____

_____

_____

_____

_____

_____

Don't play *RUSSIAN ROULETTE* with your health.

My health journey   Date_____

_____

_____

_____

_____

_____

_____

_____

_____

_____

_____

_____

_____

_____

_____

_____

_____

_____

Healthy food choices might be expensive, but illness will *COST YOU* more.

My health journey Date_____

_____

_____

_____

_____

_____

_____

_____

_____

_____

_____

_____

_____

_____

_____

_____

_____

_____

_____

Don't be a *DEAD MAN/WOMAN WALKING*. Invest in your
health.

My health journey

_____

_____

_____

_____

_____

_____

_____

_____

_____

_____

_____

_____

_____

_____

_____

_____

_____

_____

Looking good on the outside should be *A REFLECTION* of how you look on the inside.

My health journey

_____

_____

_____

_____

_____

_____

_____

_____

_____

_____

_____

_____

_____

_____

_____

_____

_____

_____

_____

_____

LOOKING GOOD should not be more important than *FEELING GOOD.* If you feel good, you will look good.

My health journey　　　　　　　　　Date_____

_____

_____

_____

_____

_____

_____

_____

_____

_____

_____

_____

_____

_____

_____

_____

_____

_____

A WAKE-UP CALL should not be the reason you choose to be healthy. Choose health today!

My health journey　　　　　　　　　　Date_____

_____

_____

_____

_____

_____

_____

_____

_____

_____

_____

_____

_____

_____

_____

_____

_____

_____

_____

_____

The *WISEST* investment you will ever make, is in your health.

My health journey

_____

_____

_____

_____

_____

_____

_____

_____

_____

_____

_____

_____

_____

_____

_____

_____

_____

_____

How much would you be willing to pay to *REGAIN YOUR HEALTH*? Don't lose it in the first place!

My health journey

_____

_____

_____

_____

_____

_____

_____

_____

_____

_____

_____

_____

_____

_____

_____

_____

_____

_____

_____

You say *"SOMEDAY I WILL CHANGE"*. Someday is not a day of the week. Make health your choice today.

My health journey   Date_____

_____

_____

_____

_____

_____

_____

_____

_____

_____

_____

_____

_____

_____

_____

_____

_____

_____

_____

TODAY is the only day that you have; tomorrow is not promised.
Choose health today!

My health journey

Date_____

_____

_____

_____

_____

_____

_____

_____

_____

_____

_____

_____

_____

_____

_____

_____

_____

_____

_____

_____

_____

SUCCESSFUL PEOPLE have successful habits. Healthy people
have healthy habits.

My health journey Date_____

_____

_____

_____

_____

_____

_____

_____

_____

_____

_____

_____

_____

_____

_____

_____

_____

Every human being is the author of his own health or disease.
- The Buddha.

My health journey

Date_____

_____

_____

_____

_____

_____

_____

_____

_____

_____

_____

_____

_____

_____

_____

_____

_____

_____

_____

_____

Tell me what you eat, and I will tell you *WHO YOU ARE*. - Jean
Anthelme Brillat-Savarin

My health journey   Date_____

_____

_____

_____

_____

_____

_____

_____

_____

_____

_____

_____

_____

_____

_____

_____

_____

_____

_____

Don't dig your *GRAVE* with your *TEETH*.

My health journey

_____

_____

_____

_____

_____

_____

_____

_____

_____

_____

_____

_____

_____

_____

_____

_____

_____

_____

_____

Health is more than what you eat, it's also **WHAT'S EATING YOU**. Pay attention to your thoughts and emotions.

My health journey   Date_____

_____

_____

_____

_____

_____

_____

_____

_____

_____

_____

_____

_____

_____

_____

_____

_____

_____

Everything that you need to be healthy is already within you.
Renew your mind and your body will follow.

My health journey
Date_____

_____

_____

_____

_____

_____

_____

_____

_____

_____

_____

_____

_____

_____

_____

_____

_____

_____

What you eat becomes *YOUR BLOOD*, your cells, and your tissues. Life is in the blood. Choose life today.

My health journey

_____

_____

_____

_____

_____

_____

_____

_____

_____

_____

_____

_____

_____

_____

_____

_____

_____

_____

_____

Press the reverse button if you are not happy with your health.
Only you have the power to change.

My health journey

Date_____

_____

_____

_____

_____

_____

_____

_____

_____

_____

_____

_____

_____

_____

_____

_____

_____

_____

_____

The journey of a thousand miles begins with a single step. - Lao Tzu.